I0414258

Anti-Inflammatory Diet

The Ultimate way to Heal yourself faster with Food, Restore Overall Health and Become Pain Free (With 1 FULL Month Meal Plan to Eliminate Pain, Increase Your Health and Aid Weight Loss!)

By:

Martin McGrann

Published by Shepal Publishing
All Rights Reserved
Copyright 2016, New York

Table of Contents

Chapter 1:
Anti-Inflammation Diet Basics

How much do you control your inflammation? You would be amazed to discover that you control a large amount of it, by the way that you treat your body, your overall health and the foods that you consume. If you have an inflammatory condition, or know someone who does, this book will be a real page turner. If you do not have these issues, prepare to expand your knowledge on anti-inflammation foods, and how they can transform a lifestyle faster than normal medicine.

First, you need to understand what the results of this diet will be. You will find that you have reduced inflammation, elevated your energy levels, and filled the body with rich nutrients that facilitate optimal functioning.

Second, you must be familiar with the rules of this diet as they are different from any other that you have tried. The principles of this diet are as follows: -

- Your daily calorie intake (for an adult) will be no less than 2000 calories a day. At the most, you can consume 3000 calories. If you are not very active, you may need to consume even less calories on a daily basis, and it is worth noting that men will need to take in much more calories than women. When you are consuming the right amount of calories based on your level of activity, you will not experience any issues with your body weight.

- You will increase your intake of water substantially. Even though you do not drink water directly, you will make room for drinking abundant amounts of tea, having lemon slices in sparkling water, or drinking juice that has been diluted.

- Your balanced meal shall change. Four main components will make up your meals. Carbohydrates consumption will be between 160 and 300 grams on a daily basis. As with most healthy meal plans, ensure that the carbohydrates are whole foods and not refined in any way.

Then there is a certain amount of fat that you can consume on this diet, although you must make sure that it is the right fat. You have approximately 67 grams of daily fat. Fatty fish which are excellent sources of omega 3 fatty acids should be consumed. You will cut back on anything that contains fat which has been saturated.

You will also be consuming protein on this diet, aiming to reach at most 120 grams each day. The type of protein that you consume is important, and it is recommended that you prioritize plant proteins. If you want to consume animal protein, opt for cheese, natural yoghurt or good quality first.

The fourth component is fiber, which will call for elevated consumption of raw vegetables and fruits. On average, you will need to take in at least forty grams of fiber on a daily basis. Most of the fiber that you consume will come from vegetables and fruits, as well as a range of cereals.

When you put all of your food on a plate, you should have a serving that is approximately 40% of carbohydrates, 30% of protein and another 30% of fat.

- Another essential part of the anti-inflammatory diet is the consumption of phytonutrients. You will find this in some plants which are meant to be of great advantage to human health. These will also help to keep certain diseases at bay. Mushrooms and vegetables will have these nutrients. When choosing your vegetables, make sure that they have a considerable amount of color, especially bright colors and dark greens.

  You can also consume reasonable amounts of tea, rather than taking in any coffee. Red wine in small doses is also a good idea, as is plain dark chocolate.

- It is important that your body receives all the minerals and vitamins that it needs. While on this diet, it is recommended that you take a multi-vitamin supplement, as well as a multi-mineral one. To ensure that the supplements are able to perform at peak, they should be consumed just before the main daily meals.

- Water is an ingredient that many people take for granted, but when you drink it you will find that it has an excellent effect on your inflammation. You can drink water in various forms, including in herbal teas, juice that has been diluted, or even sparkling with a slice of lemon within it. You should make sure that the water you consume does not have any chlorine within it.

So far, this diet does not sound too challenging because you are able to consume a range of foods, including all the food groups, and your daily calorie count is not too low, However, when you consider the types of foods that are typical of the American diet, you will understand why some would find it a challenge. It takes on an approach that is much more traditional and Mediterranean, in that you will need to consume foods which are much more wholesome, like whole grains, vegetables, fruits and beans. If you want to experience much less pain from inflammation, you are guaranteed to do so.

There are certain things that can help make this diet easier to follow, as well as more effective. One of these is paying attention to the colors of the fruits and vegetables that you are consuming. It is best to consume a range of colors each day. This means that you should have your rich greens, such as avocado and spinach, bright yellows from bananas and star fruit, orange from carrots and oranges, red from tomatoes and berries and so on. It is the bright colored foods that are recognized as having elevated anti-inflammatory benefits.

Chapter 2:
Heal your Body and Forget Inflammation

Inflammation is a signal that something is not right within your body. For you to be aware that there is an area which is inflamed, a message is sent to your brain so that you can get uncomfortable or feel pain. When you do not deal with the inflammation, this message continues being sent consistently until the pain that you are feeling becomes unbearable. For you to reduce the pain that you feel, you need a lasting solution, the best of which is the anti-inflammatory diet.

There are two types of inflammation that cause problems, and these are chronic inflammation and acute inflammation. When inflammation is acute, it is short term in nature, but, that also means that it happens very quickly and can be quite intense. On the other hand, when it is chronic, it develops over a long period of time, sometimes taking years before ravaging the body. If you have problems with inflammation, the more you ignore it or let it be without taking steps to combat, the further you will be from enjoying your life and leaving without pain.

When you have inflammation that is chronic, the tissues that are within your body are unable to heal well. On the outside, you will notice that the area that has not healed is swelling and is red in color. On the inside, you may feel some warmth or heat, and pain. This type of inflammation is more likely to remain within your body for a long time.

There are numerous illnesses that this diet is able to affect directly. On this diet, you will find that you have less pain and you save yourself from suffering with acute inflammation. These illnesses include the following: -

- Tonsillitis

- Sinusitis

- Bronchitis

- Meningitis

- Dermatitis

- Appendicitis

- Infected ingrown toenail

- Sore throat from a flu

- Broken skin from a scratch

When you have these diseases and they are acute in nature, you will find that this diet will transform your experience, helping to heal you from the inside.

For chronic inflammation, you may suffer from the following ailments: -

- Rheumatoid Arthritis

- Cancers

- Alzheimer's

- Chronic active hepatitis

- Heart Disease

- Obesity

- Chronic sinusitis

- Tuberculosis

- Chronic peptic ulcer

- Asthma

In addition to these diseases, you may develop chronic inflammation as a result of elevated stress, not maintain a good level of fitness, or consuming foods which fill your body with dangerous toxins. Although you may choose to handle the symptoms of these conditions by consuming various prescriptions medications, these do not offer long term solutions. They simply help to handle the symptoms on the surface, without truly dealing with the core issue. Changing your diet is not only more sustainable, it is also more natural.

Within this book, you will find that there are a large number of nutrients that will help you to bring down your inflammation. Nonetheless, your starting point should always be a healthy diet. This is because your body needs to have the right nutrients so that it is able to function properly. Take for example a diet that cuts out all carbohydrates in an attempt to make sure that you lose weight. This will not be effective as it will actually lead to the promotion of your inflammation. You need to have those carbohydrates within you if you want to make sure that you have the energy that is necessary.

When you eat healthily, you will have all the calories that you need to actually result in long lasting and sustainable weight loss. Make sure that you are consuming a fair amount of vegetables and fruits so that you are able to get the right amount of fiber, which will help you stay full. These kind of foods also keep your calorie intake down. In addition, the consumption of whole grains will also make sure that you remain fuller for longer. If you want to consume any dairy products, you should ensure that they are free of fat or low in fat. Consuming the food that is right will ensure that you are able to manage your condition, and live your life free of any pain. This is why you need to ensure that you fully understand what is happening in the anti-inflammatory diet.

When you consider that the anti-inflammation diet will help to ease your suffering and elevate your health, you will begin to realize the amazing benefits that it offers to you and the quality of your life. Even if you are not suffering from inflammation and pain, you need this diet to help maintain your good health. Inflammation starts within you, and by the time that you can physically tell from the outside it may have escalated into a big issue. So in addition to this diet being a partial cure for your condition, it is also excellent for prevention.

Chapter 3:
Inflammation and Weight Loss

There are a large number of complications with your health that occur as a result of being overweight, and having more weight than necessary is a trigger for inflammation. What happens is that the extra fats that you have within you are store up like active tissues. This leads to the production of certain hormones in unbalanced amounts. Therefore, if you want to reduce inflammation within your body, you can begin by bringing down your weight considerably. This should be the case if you are overweight. Should you be underweight, you must consider other alternative.

The process of weight reduction should not be sudden and drastic, Rather, you need to take it gradually, and you will find that you begin to see reduction in your inflammation faster than you could have imagined. Here are some tips to you with this.

- Keep yourself active – On this diet, you do not need to suddenly begin going to the gym for several hours in the day. What you need to do is take some time to do exercises on a daily basis. By walking for half an hour, you are keeping your entire body fit, helping with your circulation, burning your excess calories and supporting your healthy eating efforts.

- Enjoy your Food – One factor that causes people to fail when pursuing meal plans is the pressure that comes with eating foods that you do not like, for long periods of time. When the diet ends, binge eating of your favorite foods destroys your results. On this diet, you learn how to make excellent substitutions, so that you can still enjoy your favorite meals, with lower calories, higher fiber and more goodness. For example, you can make delicious ice-cream with a blended banana, or you can have soya milk instead of dairy. You are also allowed the occasional treat, including a small piece of dark chocolate to help unwind after a long day.

- No More Red Meat – From the get go, you need to understand and accept that you will no longer be consuming red meat. Your main animal protein will come from fish, and you can consume all types of fish, especially the fatty fish. If this seems like a tall order, you can treat yourself with a cheat day for some red meat in one meal, once, every fortnight. Or, you could set some goals, and when you meet these goals, you reward yourself with a little red meat. You can motivate yourself in this way, and over time, you will find that you do not need to consume red meat at all.

- Fiber is important

  Many diets will focus on your carbohydrate, fat and protein intake, with minimal attention paid to fiber. On this diet, you need to always have fiber in mind, at every meal you are consuming. You can get the fiber that you need by eating lots of vegetables and fruits, and ensuring that anything you snack on has some fiber as well. The anti-inflammation properties that fiber will include should not be underestimated.

There is one major food item that you need to consume on the anti-inflammation diet so that you can reduce your weight, and also your inflammation. That is water. You need to drink a minimum of eight glasses of water on a daily basis, but aim to reach at least double of that amount. This means that you will be drinking water from morning to evening. Also ensure that in any beverage that you are drinking, the focus is on water.

Chapter 4:
Choosing the Right
Anti-Inflammatory Foods

Inflammation is normally appreciated, until it gets to the point that it spirals out of control and causes you acute pain. There are foods that will make inflammation much worse than it should be and those foods include sugars and saturated fats. When combined with the stress and strain of daily life, as well as the toxins that are within our environment, it becomes key to limit the chances of inflammation by consuming the 'right' foods. When you do so, you fight more than inflammation, and can positively affect your chances of developing heart disease, memory loss, cancer, muscular degeneration and strokes.

As you go through the foods that you should be consuming, you may be amazed at the number of foods that you should avoid which are a part of your daily diet. Foods that have a large amount of saturated fats are not good, as are certain types of sugar, particularly those that have been processed extensive. These are the types of foods that you need to avoid.

Here are the foods that you need to consume.

Whole Grains

You will not be consuming processed flours during this diet, as whole grains are better for your inflammation. This means that refined foods, such as cereal, rice, white flour and pasta are off the menu. Whole grains have more fiber, which is what your body needs. When your body has this fiber, it is able to bring down the levels of a reactive protein in Vitamin C that is known for increases inflammation within your blood. As you are purchasing foods that have been labeled as whole grain, read the label carefully to ensure that there is no added sugar.

Fatty Fish

These are the type of fish that are not typically white in color of their flesh. They are normally oily in nature, and include tuna, sardines, salmon and mackerel. These types of fish have elevated levels of Omega 3 fatty acids, that have been proven to be highly effective when dealing with inflammation.

For the best results, they need to be consumed at least for times in a week. The preparation method used for this fish is key, and baking them, grilling or boiling have the best results.

Low Fat Dairy

On this diet, you can consume dairy products, though they need to be low in fat to bring down your inflammation. They will also help to improve your levels of protein in the body. The best that you can consume is yoghurt, which is rich in inflammation reducing probiotics. In addition, your body will benefit from Vitamin D and calcium.

Leafy Vegetables

All leafy vegetables will help reduce inflammation, though the very best are those whose leaves are dark green. These would include spinach, kales, broccoli and others. These are recognized as being power houses of minerals and vitamins, and also have high doses of iron. Your body has a large number of pro-inflammatory molecules within it, and these help to combat them.

Peppers

These include the hot and chili kind. You should also have those which are the colorful and flavorful find which are also known as capsicums. You will immediately be attracted to eating them due to their bright colors and strong fragrance. These also have the benefit of containing a large amount of antioxidants, and having limited starch.

If you choose to consume chili, they will have capsaicin, which is an active ingredient that will help to bring down your overall pain. What you need to do is pay attention to how these foods are affecting your body and you will know whether or not they are helping with your inflammation.

Nuts

On this diet, you can consume foods that have fat, though you need to be careful about the type of fat you consume as saturated fats are to be avoided. Instead, go for healthy fats, such as those which you can find in nuts. Nuts are also rich in fiber and antioxidants, which are able to help the body to repair the underlying cause of your inflammation.

Ginger and Turmeric

It is possible to spice up your meals by consuming ginger and turmeric. Even the smallest doses of these spices can have a major and positive effect on your inflammation. They have properties which help the regulation of the immune system, meaning that when good inflammation is necessary, it can be triggered off faster to deal with the problem before it goes out of control.

Soy

This is a small bean that is very rich in protein and highly versatile. It contains isoflavones which are compounds that are similar to estrogen. These help to bring down the levels of inflammation. You should be careful to avoid soy which has been over processed as it will not bring about the benefits that you are hoping for. This is largely due to the fact that it will contain a significant number of preservatives, as well as additives that will cause the body more harm than good. You could consume soy milk or the beans themselves, or if you like, some tofu.

Berries

Although fruits as a whole are great for fighting inflammation, berries are known to be the best fruits you can consume in this case. They are high in antioxidants and have a chemical known anthocyanin which has excellent anti-inflammatory properties. In addition, they have the benefits of being low in calories, low in fat and low in carbohydrates. Different berries will have different benefits. For example, blue berries are known to fight inflammation within the intestines, and raspberries are known for prevention of arthritis.

Chocolate

This is one food that will put a smile on your face, as for many people, it is a favorite food. You may doubt how it will help your anti-inflammation diet considering the amount of sugar that normal chocolate will have. The key is to consume some dark chocolate as it is able to provide excellent anti-inflammatory benefits. In addition to this, it also has properties that are anti-oxidants, further extending its total health benefits. They key is to have it in moderation, and to ensure that it is at least 75% cocoa within its content.

Beetroot and Tomatoes

These are two vegetables that are rich in color. Both have antioxidants within them, Beetroot are also sources of Vitamin C and have excellent levels of fiber. They should be consumed raw in juice or grated into salads and meals. They will help with management of pain as well we the effects of inflammation.

Tomatoes contain lycopene which is able to bring down inflammation all over the body, particularly in the lungs. They will have excellent effects whether you cook them before consumption or eat them raw. What this means is that juices or condiments that contain tomatoes can be consumed and still have great effects.

Olive Oil

You will need to consume some fat while you are on this diet, so it makes sense that you ensure it is healthy fat. Olive oil is good for you, and also has properties that make it an excellent anti-inflammatory food. When choosing from the variety that you find in the market, select the extra virgin kind as this is the purest.

There is an ingredient in olive oil that fights inflammation and it is known as oleocanthal. It has benefits that are very similar to pain killers, which will make inflammation that is accompanied by pain much easier to deal with.

Choosing the right foods is an excellent step that you should take, but knowing the wrong foods is just as important. There are plenty of foods that cause inflammation but here are the ones you should keep away from or minimize as much as possible.

Eggs

These are present in a variety of dishes and loved by many because they are high in protein. Eggs can cause inflammation if you have an allergy to them in any way. If you are troubled with inflammation, remove eggs from your diet for a few weeks and see what the effects may be. If your symptoms disappear, keep these out of your diet. If they do not, then you can eat your eggs, though make sure you do so in moderation.

Wheat

Like eggs, you will find that in a day you consume a large amount of products that have wheat. These include staples like pasta, and also baked goods like cakes and cookies. You should avoid foods that contain wheat and choose others which are similar but are less inflammatory. These will often have the added benefit of being lower in overall carbohydrates as well. Some people experience inflammation because of gluten, so cutting out wheat also gets rid of these problems.

Certain Fruits

You are encouraged to eat fruits while on this diet, yet there are certain fruits that you need to avoid as you may be sensitive to them. These fruits include the citrus variety, such as lemons and oranges. There are other fruits that are problematic, including mangoes, pineapples and papayas. Keeping away from them is the ideal solution for anyone looking to avoid inflammation.

Meat that is Not Organic

Organic meat does not contain any chemicals but inorganic meat is full of dangerous ingredients. These are the types of foods which cause inflammation, and will negatively affect your health. You need meat in your diet in order to get the right levels of proteins, so make sure that you are choosing the right meats for the success of your diet.

These are some of the foods that can help you powerfully reduce your inflammation, as they are rich in antioxidants, vitamins and minerals that your body needs. When consuming anything, you should make sure it is as close to its natural form as possible. Cutting out all processed foods is essential, as is eating as much raw food as possible. Look for foods that are labelled as organic to ensure that you are not harming your efforts by loading your body with unnecessary chemicals. While on this diet, you need to cut out all alcohol as well, as this burdens your liver and affects it ability to remove toxins from your body.

Chapter 5:
4 Week Meal Plan

The anti-inflammation diet is not about excessive restrictions to your diet. Instead, you should view it as a diet that enables you to take control of your meals, your inflammation and your life. In a period of four weeks, you can make a considerable difference to what is happening within your body, and lose weight, improve your healthy as well as get rid of any plan. This diet plan consists of a meal plan for four weeks, and information on how to maintain the diet.

Some tips for you to remember include: -

- Four servings of fruit and five servings of vegetables each day.

- Whole meal pasta or brown rice three times a week.

- No less that two servings of fish in a week.

- More plant protein than animal protein consumption each week.

- Dietary supplements including Vitamins C, D and E, Carotenoids, Selenium and Calcium each day.

Week One – Getting Started

There are two things that you will be doing in addition to eating specific foods in this week. These are getting clear about what is happening within your body, and making a commitment that will last you're a lifetime. Although this is a four-week plan, it is expected that at the end of this time period, you will be able to stay on this diet for the rest of your life.

So begin by taking stock of your vital statistics. Measure out your body using a tape measure, and also check on your weight. Start keeping a log of your sleep on an average day. Make the necessary cuts from your diet by cleaning out your kitchen cupboards. This means that you need to get rid of processed foods and anything else that could cause you to go off course with this diet.

After you have dealt with yourself physically, and your environment, you need to look at where you are emotionally. List down the things that you consider motivational and why you want to follow through with this diet plan. Having clear motives will make it easier for you to meet your goals.

Incorporate 30 minutes of exercise into your daily routine, and ensure that each night you are able to sleep for eight hours. During the day, you will be consuming a total of five meals. There shall be three main meals, and two snacks. Allocate a fixed time for your meal consumption so that you create a pattern for your body to follow.

At each meal, you will be consuming fruit or vegetables, either whole, juiced or as smoothies. Your beverages will consist of water and green tea, and you will gradually cut coffee from your diet. Here is a meal plan that will help to guide you for the first seven days. Make your choice of meals that you will repeat on the weekend.

Choose from the following breakfast dishes

1. Oatmeal and Banana, Green Tea and Spinach Smoothie

2. Fruit Slices with Chia Seeds, Natural Yoghurt, and ½ teaspoon almonds

3. Sliced peaches with sprinkling of ground cinnamon, Carrot Juice

4. Tropical fruit salad

5. Banana, Coconut and Walnut Mix

Choose from the following mid-morning snacks

1. One tablespoon almonds

2. One tablespoon walnuts

3. One tablespoon pistachios

4. Mixed berries salad

5. Whole meal and Oat Muffin

All mid-morning snacks to be accompanied with a cup of green tea.

Choose from the following lunch dishes

1. Grilled Tuna Steak, Green salad with vinaigrette, Watermelon

2. Mixed Vegetable Soup, Green Salad with Vinaigrette

3. Avocado Salad with Vinaigrette, Papaya

4. Steamed Chicken and Vegetables in Whole Meal Wrap, Apple

5. Smoked Salmon and Green Salad with Vinaigrette, Orange

Choose from the following mid-afternoon snacks

1. Veggie sticks and almond butter

2. Rye Crackers with Avocado

3. Mixed berry smoothie

4. Whole meal and Blueberry Muffin.

5. Celery sticks and peanut butter

Choose from the following dinner dishes

1. Brown Rice and Vegetable Curry

2. Turkey Meatballs, whole meal Spaghetti, Steamed Spinach and Mango

3. Sweet Potato, Bean Chili and Whole meal flat bread, Green Salad and Mango

4. Salmon cakes and Cauliflower, with apple

5. Mexican Beans, Avocado Salad, Banana

Week Two –
Staying on Track

By the time you have completed the first week, you should be have overcome a range of cravings that you have, and started seeing food in a new way. Nonetheless, you are still vulnerable to triggers that could cause you to fall of course. Therefore, you need to find a way that you can fight these temptations, while staying on course.

First, you need to allow yourself a special day each week, where you can have a cheat food. This is not a day to indulge in bad eating, but a day where you allow yourself one treat, such as a biscuit. This treat will not damage all your efforts, but should help you satisfy a physical and psychological craving.

Your intensity in exercise should increase as well, as you move up your session from thirty minutes to forty-five. Sleep remains the same eight hours, and meals also remain fixed. When it comes to the menu, you can start to become a little more flexible, ensuring that you are staying in line with consuming fruits and vegetables through the day. When you find that you are hungry, keep some grapes or blueberries close by, and snack on these instead of something else that would be unhealthy. In case you do not have enough time to create your own menu, here is are some food options to consider.

Choose from the following breakfast dishes

1. Wholegrain Toast, Boiled Egg and fresh cherries

2. Oat porridge with mixed berries

3. Banana, Coconut and Walnut Mix

4. Tropical Fruit Salad

5. Millet porridge with coconut and bananas

Choose from the following mid-morning snacks

1. Hummus with assorted veggie sticks

2. Mixed berries topped with natural yoghurt

3. Peanut butter and celery sticks

4. Whole meal muffin

5. Mixed vegetable broth, Coleslaw Salad with Vinaigrette dressing, Banana

All mid-morning snacks to be accompanied with a cup of green tea.

Choose from the following lunch dishes

1. Whole meal Spinach Lasagna

2. Beetroot and Carrot Salad, Mango

3. Chicken and Green Salad Wrap

4. Sardines, lemon and herb salad with vinaigrette

5. Apple, broccoli and cranberry salad with vinaigrette

Choose from the following mid-afternoon snacks

1. Banana Smoothie

2. Mango Smoothie

3. Kale and Spinach Smoothie

4. Pineapple and Ginger smoothie

5. Watermelon Smoothie

Choose from the following dinner dishes

1. Ginger and Garlic Steamed Trout, Carrot Puree and Green Salad

2. Vegetable Soup and an Apple

3. Grilled Salmon with sautéed mushrooms, quinoa and Steamed Vegetables

4. Trout and Ginger steamed, with garlic sweet potato mash, Banana

5. Turkey meatballs, steamed spinach and whole meal pasta

Week Three –
Handle your Physical and Emotional Environments

A serious and often neglected cause of inflammation is stress, which affects what happens to you physically as well as emotionally. Now that you are getting your body to view foods in a different way, you do not want to sabotage your efforts by having your mind work against you. Look at any activities in your life that may be causing your stress and deal with them. As you support your efforts with exercises as well as sleeping for the right number of hours each night, you will find that you can get great results and reduce your inflammation considerably. Here is a plan to help with your food consumption this week.

Choose from the following breakfast dishes

1. Millet Porridge and Blueberries

2. Muesli

3. Blueberries, Quinoa and Toasted Walnuts

4. Oatmeal and Banana, Green Tea

5. Fruit platter with coconut and almonds

Choose from the following mid-morning Snacks

1. Banana and Cinnamon Smoothie

2. Watermelon Smoothie

3. One teaspoon of pistachios

4. Whole meal and Oat Muffin

5. Celery Sticks with Peanut Butter

All mid-morning snacks to be accompanied with a cup of green tea.

Choose from the following lunch dishes

1. Grilled Salmon, Spinach Salad with Vinaigrette, Banana

2. Beetroot and Carrot Salad, Mango

3. Tuna and Green Salad Wrap

4. Bean Burger with whole meal bun, Green Salad and Vinaigrette

5. Apple, broccoli and cranberry salad with vinaigrette

Choose from the following mid-afternoon snacks

1. One teaspoon of almonds

2. One teaspoon of Walnuts

3. Kale and Spinach Smoothie

4. Hummus and Veggie sticks

5. Pineapple and Ginger smoothie

Choose from the following dinner dishes

1. Lentil Curry with Brown Rice, Orange

2. Mushroom Soup and an Apple

3. Grilled Chicken Breast, Avocado Salad and Steamed Vegetables

4. Tofu stuffed wholegrain wrap, Green salad

5. Mixed vegetable broth, Coconut and Bananas

Week Four –
Change your Life

In this week, you will put in place systems to help you adopt a healthy eating meal plan for the rest of your life. Fighting inflammation is not like fighting a fire. When you put out the flames in a fire, you have essentially destroyed it, but with inflammation, you would only have temporarily destroyed the fire. A spark could remain, reigniting another fire unless it is properly dealt with.

Now you know the types of meals that you should be consuming, so you can create a plan that works for you in this week. Go through all your kitchen cupboards again one more time, and get rid of any processed foods that are within them, including things like soda and sugar. Purchase substitutes of these products. Make sure that any carbohydrates you consume are brown. Finally, if you do not live alone, recruit the rest of your family on your healthy eating plan, as supporting each other to transforming your lifestyles will make it possible to experience amazing benefits both in reducing your inflammation and dealing with a host of other health issues.

Chapter 6:
Tips to Keep You Going

At any time that you are looking to change your diet, you will realize the difficulty you can experience when you are moving away from habits, particularly if these habits revolve around food that is healthy. Many people find it challenging to stay on track with the diet plan, even when they know that they are risking their overall health. If this is you on the anti-inflammatory diet, then you are not alone and there are some tips that can make the process for you much easier.

Get the Support You Need

When you have made the decision to start on this diet, make sure that you have a support system in place. People who support you through this process will make it easier for you follow through with your plans. When you have a good system of support, you will find that it is much easier for you to combat your cravings and build your health.

Maintain a Food Journal

You need to be able to keep track of what you are eating, and the best way to do so is a food journal. However, make sure that your food journal is much richer than this in regards to information. Also include information on your feelings, especially what you feel when you are having a craving. This way, you will identify your triggers, and also keep track of what works for you to minimize them. With a journal, you can have a plan that is long term in nature so that you do not affect your health.

Get Adventurous

Preparing the same meals each day is the simplest way to end up breaking your routine due to monotony. Instead, you need to look for a range of recipes that are much more fun, making use of herbs and spices as much as you can. Make sure that you are always looking for new recipes that you can try, especially those which are tasty.

Get Together with Friends

Often times when people are on a diet, they tend to avoid their friends and social activities so that they can keep away from temptation. If you are fighting inflammation, there is no need for you to stop having a good time and keep away from being social. You can do some things to help you resist temptation. For example, before you go out with your friends for dinner, have something to eat while you are at home. Then, when you are out, you may end up looking to eat a salad or something simple and light as well. You still get to enjoy the company of your peers, without worry that you are falling off the wagon. Do not keep your diet a secret. Let your friends know as well so that they can support you where possible.

Eat Fresh Food

For this diet to be successful, you need to eat as much fresh food in your diet as possible. This is because foods which are fresh will have more benefits to your health than any other. In addition to being more tasty, they will also have more vibrant colors and better appeal. Make sure that you cut out as much processed food as possible. Processed foods will also lack in fiber, and in the long run, will not be good for your overall health.

With these tips, you will experience a transformation of both the mind and the body when on the anti-inflammation diet. You will find it easy to extend this diet beyond a month, and make it a part of your long term plan in life. A change in lifestyle is what you need to improve your long term quality of life.

Conclusion

When you have inflammation, your body suffers as a result, and you may bring about a range of diseases which are purely related to your health. On this diet, you will be able to manage the symptoms and fill your body with what it needs to fight inflammation effectively.

The anti-inflammation diet is more than a diet, as it is a journey that will lead to an amazing change in your life. What you want is lasting change, so you need to give this diet time to feel its effects. Do not give up if you do not see some results within the first two weeks. Keep up the effort and you will be glad that you did so.

Remember, it is all about choosing alternatives so that you can recreate your favorite meals, with higher levels of nutrients. The more you choose this natural way of managing your inflammation, the less you will depend on conventional prescribed medication in the long run.